Archangel 101

COMMUNICATION & DIVINATION GUIDEBOOK

Lisa Nicole

Archangel 101

Communication & Divination

Guidebook

By Lisa Nicole
Copyright © 2018. Lisa Nicole
All rights reserved.

ISBN: 9781791685836

First Edition 2018

Printed in the United States of America

Dedication:

This book is dedicated to the REAL you. The YOU that is ready and waiting to be revealed.

Table of Contents

Experiencing the vast variety of unique vibrations of the many different Angels is wonderful and completely fascinating, in my opinion! Meeting the Archangels can change your life, it sure changed mine. I'm thrilled to tell you more about some of my personal angelic experiences during this chapter & through interactive online course experience , that I offer as well.

I want to be clear and say the Angels are just an extension of you. They are not outside of you or above you. Angelic awareness operates on a high level of frequency. We each have a unique frequency and vibrational imprint. Your unique blend of vibrational frequencies makes up YOU. There is a Higher Intelligence that resides in the outmost & innermost parts of ALL of Us, of all of our Souls. That Higher Source has condensed itself to make it possible for all experience, for us to be Souls. The Archangels are like the ingredients & attributes of the Higher Self, Higher Source. Imagine a decadent & grand 12 tiered wedding cake made up of every delectable ingredient & decoration available. Imagine those same ingredients uniquely combined in a smaller, individual recipes & versions of the masterpiece. You are that cupcake, the Archangels represent the ingredients, uniquely combined in each of us. When you call upon an the Archangel you are calling upon the part of you, that attribute within yourself that IS that. A concentrated version of THAT. This Guidebook Course is meant to a a fun and great way to access these inner parts of you, and your gifts through your own experiences.

*Love at first sight: I personally opened up to the Archangels when I began to walk through the path of healing my own **Thyroid Disease**, even though I was told it would never happen, by a doctor. In 2011, I was diagnosed with Hashimoto's. This was after the 11 month battle of my life. That's whole book in itself. Auto -immune issues & diseases can be managed. It's common for those of us who are sensitive and intuitively tuned in mohave issue sin this area. My biggest contributor to healing was & is Archangel Raphael, my dear friend & trusted companion, who helped lead me through the process of self-healing through the process of self love. This was the beginning of the awareness to my awakening. So, I ask what is leading you here? To this journey amongst Angels? The Angels are your family. Your Mind, Body & Soul is calling to be honored. You've answered that call. Well done. For me, with he Angels, it was love at first sight.*

Archangels are omnipresent. They can be everywhere, all at once. They can be in more than one place at time.

There are a few Angels that I communicate with on a regular basis, and a limitless amount of them to connect with at any given time. We will explore YOUR personal connection in this guidebook, Archangel 101. I also ask that you leave your knowledge, Sunday school teachings, family traditions and rituals at the door. Leave your ancient text and passed down stories of childhood aside. We are writing our own ancient text of the future. Here and now. Let so that with fresh perspectives and open minds. Be open to viewing that new perspective, in this space, you are safe to explore new ideas. Like window shopping, only buy what you love and what fits. You can simply view, and return to your original belief or concept at anytime. If something does not resonate for you, don't buy it. Like leaving your coat checked at the door, you can always pick it up when you are done.

There has been a lot written about Archangels in many of the ancient texts, I want you to feel them, for yourself. Your experience, your connection. Learning to trust your own inner knowledge & wisdom. Several stories and ideas have been passed along as Truth by many religious organizations and other contributors. If you have a preconceived notion of Angels, I am here asking you to set all of that concept or idea aside, for the purpose of this experience.

My personal relationship with the energy of the Archangels is not that of a religious one, in case you hadn't picked up on that yet. I was not raised in any particular religion or faith. I was raised on Love & Trust. I was fortunate enough to have a mostly non-biased idea of what the the Archangels are and what they represent. The only Angel in my life was the one on top of a Christmas tree every year.

I could talk about the Angels for days, and we can, in the FB group and course videos! I really don't want to give you too much background or information on them here, I want it to be yours not what Iv'e told you. Might sound completely silly not to give a lot of info, since this is a book on the Archangels, right? Listen, you can Google anything you like on them. There's lots of "standard" or "common" info on many of the Archangel. That being said your interpretation may be totally doffing for the rest of the the World, and that's ok. Trust YOU, always. There are factoids all over the place on the internet that you can read on Michael or Raphael. I'm not here to throw factoids at you, though. You will find some clues sprinkled within the lines of this guidebook. I am here to hold and create space for YOU to connect on your own! My mission is to give you the opportunity , that I was given. I want you to open up to MORE, I want you to find what you SEEK in your HEART. I wish for you to find your place in the family of the Archangels, just like I have.

> **~ Do you already talk to the Archangels?**
> **~ Do they talk or communicate back to you?**
> **~ Maybe through music or signs?**
> **~ Do you ever see flashes of color?**

When we begin or pursue our personal path of self-healing, we are surrounded by support. These amazing beings can really assist in grand ways. In this Guidebook you will find many Angel Invocations and Intentions, these are tools to call in the Angel Energy. These invocations can be used at any time, not just for journaling or when you are in trouble or chaos! Dailey interaction with Archangels is what we are creating a sacred space for.

We are made of powerful vibrant energy, Divinely Intelligent & Infinite Energy . If we learn to access, clear, maintain and master our energetic makeup then we can create our reality and outcomes with clarity and precision. Once we grasp that energy works, creates & flows we can direct those concepts with intention. We must understand that OUR OWN CHOICES mold our reality & outcomes, WE choose bad choices that create bad outcomes. We are informed enough to responsibly shift our lives, health and perspective.

You are a Divine Being of Light and you can do anything! If you are feeling stuck, depressed, overweight, without purpose, in chronic pain, or afflicted with any disease in your body, you have the power to utilize this experience for greater purpose. You can heal, grow, and gain clarity and freedom form within. You have the power, you are the power. The Archangels are here to assist on your path of self awareness and self-healing, as am I.

You are deeply loved by the Angelic Realm and they want to talk to you. We are going to experience ways to build and strengthen that connection.

Thank you for allowing me to share my experiences and tools with you!

Essential Oils, Singing bowls, & chimes, oh my … add your unique imprint into your connection and sessions with the Archangels. Personalize your experience. Infuse your own protocol and ritual connection. I love making spray with oils & the angels. I use them in my sessions & channeling rituals.

Set your own boundaries, and rules when communicating multi-dimensionally with other beings & collectives. Regardless of "who" you are chatting it up with, YOU are always in charge.

Spiritual Toolbox 101

This is your daily spiritual toolbox, or much more like a tool **chest**. These healing tools are for you to utilize as we move through this experience. They are each to be initiated **everyday** for maximum results. These tools are to help you stay committed and organized while you go through your Angelic process. I ask that you consider adopting the use of these tools in the future, staying connected is much easier with simple routine in place. Choose what resonates with you, and commit to it as you move forward.

Please take your time working through the Guidebook. There is processing time when healing the emotional, mental & physical body. This is a process of healing through connection. Ongoing. Please be patient and allow yourself adequate space to make the most of your experience with me. I you might take some of you longer to process that others, both are perfect. Allow yourself to be guided. Listen to your body and your knowingness on when to move forward.

Calling up the energy of the Archangels during a healing session for others and for yourself, is a great way to channel their energy! Call upon their color & essence and direct it to run through you, as the channel. You may even have particular Archangels that come into your work as your Team of Healing Helpers.

As an Angel Intuitive & Ambassador of the the Light you are required to use your gifts for the betterment of ALL. Meaning, ONLY for good. You are Light & Love. Personal gain is out & manipulation of events and outcomes is prohibited.

Calling In Archangels

I like to call upon the Archangels for assistance, through meditation. I do this in the morning, before I even get out of bed. Also throughout the day, I call upon the Angels in particular situations to bring more Light.

(You may choose to recite the invocations below either aloud or mentally, both are equally as effective.)

Samples:

> *Thank you* MICHAEL *for helping me to maintain my own energy and vibration throughout the day and night. Surround my family and myself with your deep Blue Energy of Protection & Safety.*

> *Archangel* RAPHAEL, *thank you for infusing the Emerald Green Ray of healing energy into every cell of my physical body. Allowing for my own self-healing and the healing of everyone, & thing involved.*
>
> GABRIEL *I am grateful for the inner strength you highlight within me. Thank you for allowing all parties to speak their Truth with grace and ease. Communications are clear. Thank you (x3)*

> *I call upon all the entire realm of the* ARCHANGEL

*to shower me with their love and blessings. I am open to the abun-
dance of the Angelic Realm. I accept the help and support of the my
family of Archangels, thank you and so it is.(x3)*

Sit quietly, light a candle perhaps. Burn some sage & incense. Bring out your crystals and signing bowls. Maybe you'll call upon your your drum or other vibrational sound installment. Choose an essential oil to use that represent the color or virtue of the Archangel you are intending to connect with. Wear the color that matches there frequency. Use flowers that compliment there strength & virtue.

Get grounded & centered. Surrounding yourself with White Light & Love of the Highest Order. Breathing nice deep breaths.

Now, call in your Angel using an intention or invocation. Calling with your mind, telepathically. At first, It may feel like imagination. That's common. So, your doing great! Be sure to take note of how you **feel**, what you **see, hear, smell** & **think** about when you call them in and sit with their energy. Even if you hear your own voice, make note. Symbols are often times shared. You may think about a number or codes. Nothing is insignificant when connecting with and channeling energy in mediumship. Ask questions? As many as you like. Note the responses. Again you can get as detailed as you wish for your personal ritual of connection. You are creating a individual energetic form of commination with each being.

Did you know? You can utilize these methods when connecting with all spirit guides, angels, animals, plants and loved ones, here or passed on. This is mediumship.

> *Essential Oils, singing bowls, & chimes, oh my … add your unique imprint into your connection and sessions with the Archangels. Personalize your experience. Infuse your own protocol and ritual connection. I love making sprays with oils & the angels. I use them in my sessions & channeling rituals.*

> *Staying hydrated is essential when doing multi-dimensional intuitive connecting. Water is an all healing agent. Bless your water to add a extra zap of high vibrational frequency. POW!*

If you like to visualize it could be very effective for your mind eye experience. You can create a detailed backdrop in your mind. A nice curvy pathway, through a well lite forrest of pine trees, maybe. Could have streams of sunlight thought he tops of the branches and singing birds. Then at the end of the path, could be your Archangel's energy waiting for you.

Maybe you're more of a cosmic connector or traveler. Imagine you are greeted in another dimensional layer or astral plane. On another planet, ,maybe?!

You could also just…be still, and simply invite your Archangel to YOU. You may like to sit or to lay down. I fall asleep when I lay down so I like to sit up an meditate, connect, & channel.

Us this simple invocation to call in each of the Archangels.

"I invite the energy of the Archangel <u>Metatron</u> to me and through me.

Thank you. Thank you, Thank you. "

(3 X's & repeat as mantra, if necessary)

Use the sheets provided to document your experiences with each Angel.

I'd like you to work individually with each of the Archangels for at least 2

days

Archangel

Maintains & Assembles Order

Please note your experience with this Angelic Being:

What message does this energy bring?

What sights, sounds, feelings, thoughts, scents & emotions come to you?

What particular color, number or symbol has been brought to your awareness?

Archangel _______________

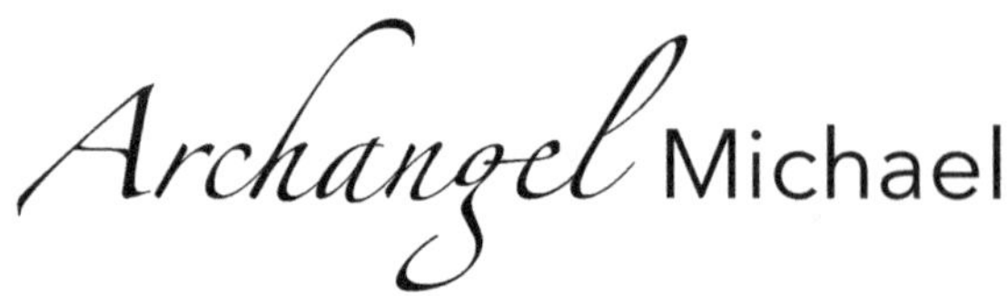

Archangel Michael

Enforcement of Clear & Subtle Boundaries

Please note your experience with this Angelic Being:

What message does this energy bring?

What sights, sounds, feelings, thoughts, scents & emotions come to you?

What particular color, number or symbol has been brought to your awareness?

Archangel

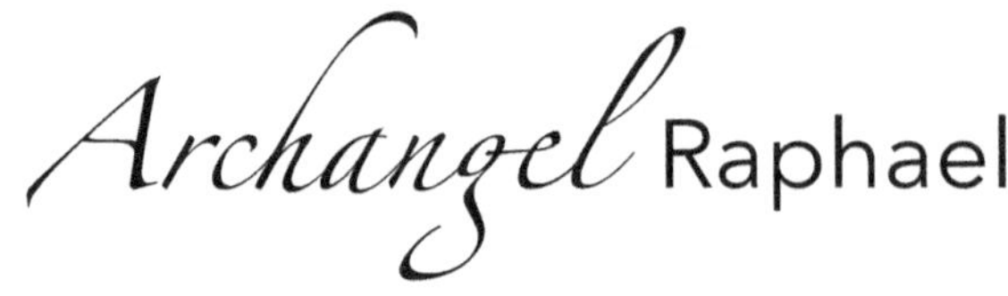# Natural Construction & Reconstruction

Please note your experience with this Angelic Being:

What message does this energy bring?

What sights, sounds, feelings, thoughts, scents & emotions come to you?

What particular color, number or symbol has been brought to your awareness?

Archangel_________

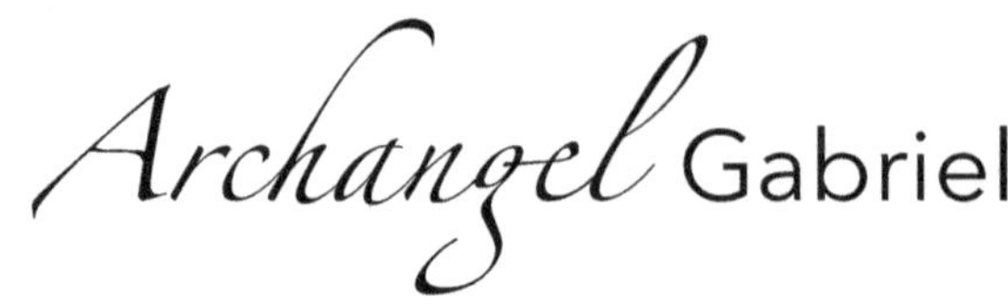

Language & Communication Programming

Please note your experience with this Angelic Being:

What message does this energy bring?

What sights, sounds, feelings, thoughts, scents & emotions come to you?

What particular color, number or symbol has been brought to your awareness?

Archangel __________

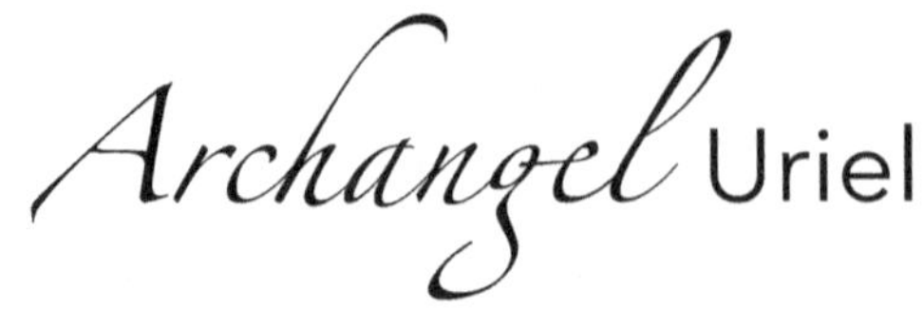

Deeply Grounded in Illumination & Wisdom

Please note your experience with this Angelic Being:

What message does this energy bring?

What sights, sounds, feelings, thoughts, scents & emotions come to you?

What particular color, number or symbol has been brought to your awareness?

Archangel__________

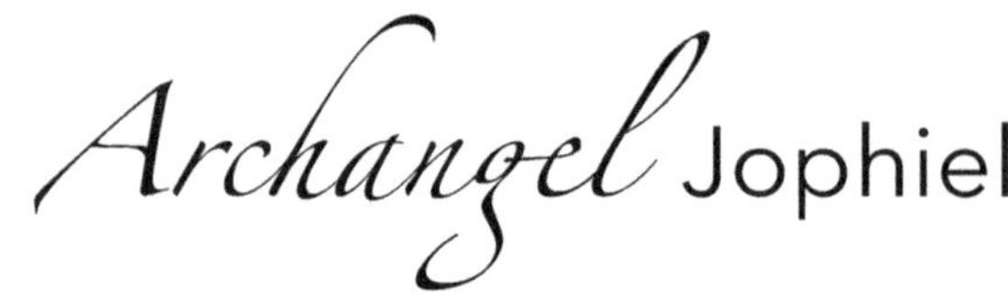

Archangel Jophiel

Creation & Beauty from Within

Please note your experience with this Angelic Being:

What message does this energy bring?

What sights, sounds, feelings, thoughts, scents & emotions come to you?

What particular color, number or symbol has been brought to your awareness?

Archangel________

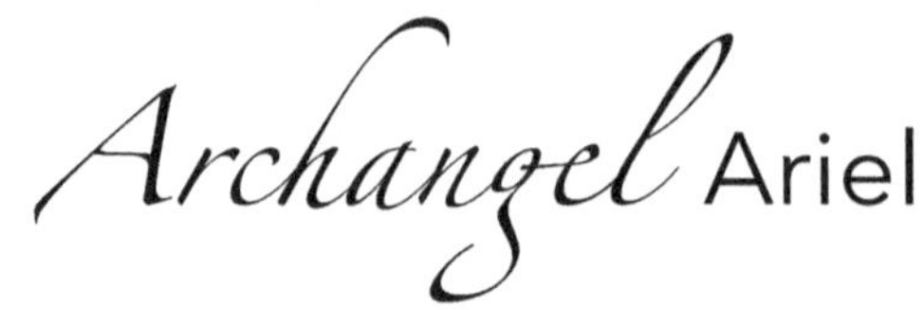

Archangel Ariel

Courage & Fortitude

Please note your experience with this Angelic Being:

What message does this energy bring?

What sights, sounds, feelings, thoughts, scents & emotions come to you?

What particular color, number or symbol has been brought to your awareness?

Archangel__________

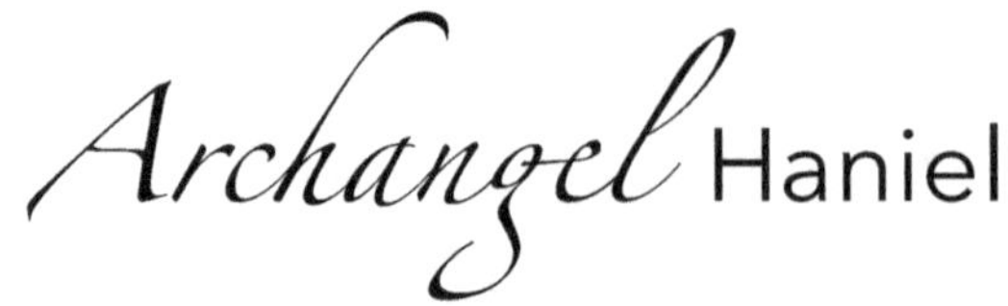

Expression of Truth & Higher Self

Please note your experience with this Angelic Being:

What message does this energy bring?

What sights, sounds, feelings, thoughts, scents & emotions come to you?

What particular color, number or symbol has been brought to your awareness?

Archangel _______

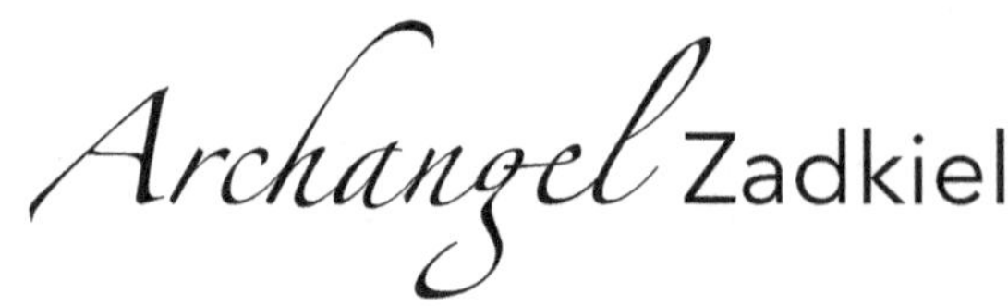

Forgiveness Resolution & Resentment Reprogramming

Please note your experience with this Angelic Being:

What message does this energy bring?

What sights, sounds, feelings, thoughts, scents & emotions come to you?

What particular color, number or symbol has been brought to your awareness?

Archangel______________

Daily Intention

I AM Grateful for

My Energy is directed

Act of Kindness

for yourself & others

Affirmation

Energy Check

Am I GROUNDED?   Y / N   Y / N

Am I HYDRATED?   Y / N   Y / N

Am I NOURISHED?   Y / N   Y / N

Archangel

Daily Intention

I AM *Grateful for*

My Energy is directed

----------→

----------→

----------→

----------→

----------→

----------→

----------→

----------→

Energy Check

Am I GROUNDED?   Y / N   Y / N

Am I HYDRATED?   Y / N   Y / N

Am I NOURISHED?   Y / N   Y / N

Act of Kindness

for yourself & others

Affirmation

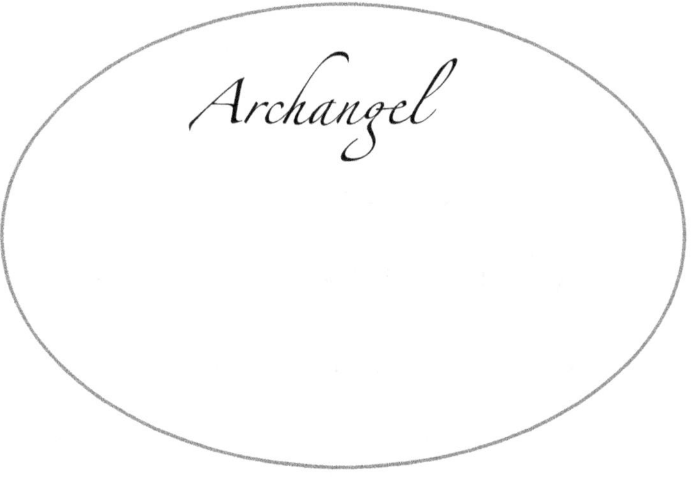

Archangel

Daily Intention

I AM *Grateful for*

My Energy is directed

Act of *Kindness*

for yourself & others

Affirmation

Energy Check

Am I GROUNDED?   Y / N   Y / N

Am I HYDRATED?   Y / N   Y / N

Am I NOURISHED?   Y / N   Y / N

Archangel

Daily Intention

I AM *Grateful for*

My Energy is directed $\longrightarrow$

- - - - - - - - - - - - - - - - ▶
- - - - - - - - - - - - - - - - ▶
- - - - - - - - - - - - - - - - ▶
- - - - - - - - - - - - - - - - ▶
- - - - - - - - - - - - - - - - ▶
- - - - - - - - - - - - - - - - ▶
- - - - - - - - - - - - - - - - ▶
- - - - - - - - - - - - - - - - ▶
- - - - - - - - - - - - - - - - ▶

Act of Kindness

for yourself & others

Affirmation

Energy Check

Am I GROUNDED?   Y / N   Y / N

Am I HYDRATED?   Y / N   Y / N

Am I NOURISHED?   Y / N   Y / N

Archangel

Daily Intention

I AM *Grateful for*

My Energy is directed ⟹

-------------------------▶
-------------------------▶
-------------------------▶
-------------------------▶
-------------------------▶
-------------------------▶
-------------------------▶
-------------------------▶
-------------------------▶

Energy Check

Am I GROUNDED?   Y / N   Y / N

Am I HYDRATED?   Y / N   Y / N

Am I NOURISHED?   Y / N   Y / N

Act of *Kindness*

for yourself & others

Affirmation

Archangel

Daily Intention

My Energy is directed →

--------→
--------→
--------→
--------→
--------→
--------→
--------→
--------→
--------→

Act of Kindness

for yourself & others

Affirmation

Energy Check

Am I GROUNDED?   Y / N   Y / N

Am I HYDRATED?   Y / N   Y / N

Am I NOURISHED?   Y / N   Y / N

Archangel

Daily Intention

I AM *Grateful for*

My Energy is directed →

→
→
→
→
→
→
→
→
→

Energy Check

Am I GROUNDED?　　Y / N　Y / N

Am I HYDRATED?　　Y / N　Y / N

Am I NOURISHED?　　Y / N　Y / N

Act of *Kindness*

for yourself & others

Affirmation

Archangel

Daily Intention

I AM Grateful for

My Energy is directed

Act of Kindness

for yourself & others

Affirmation

Energy Check

Am I GROUNDED?   Y / N   Y / N

Am I HYDRATED?   Y / N   Y / N

Am I NOURISHED?   Y / N   Y / N

Archangel

Daily Intention

I AM *Grateful for*

My Energy is directed ⟹

- - - - - - - - - - - - ➤
- - - - - - - - - - - - ➤
- - - - - - - - - - - - ➤
- - - - - - - - - - - - ➤
- - - - - - - - - - - - ➤
- - - - - - - - - - - - ➤
- - - - - - - - - - - - ➤
- - - - - - - - - - - - ➤

Energy Check

Am I GROUNDED?   Y / N Y / N

Am I HYDRATED?   Y / N Y / N

Am I NOURISHED?   Y / N Y / N

Act of Kindness

for yourself & others

Affirmation

Archangel

Daily Intention

I AM *Grateful for*

My Energy is directed

- - - - - - - - - - - - ▶
- - - - - - - - - - - - ▶
- - - - - - - - - - - - ▶
- - - - - - - - - - - - ▶
- - - - - - - - - - - - ▶
- - - - - - - - - - - - ▶
- - - - - - - - - - - - ▶
- - - - - - - - - - - - ▶

Act of Kindness

for yourself & others

Affirmation

Energy Check

Am I GROUNDED?   Y / N   Y / N

Am I HYDRATED?   Y / N   Y / N

Am I NOURISHED?   Y / N   Y / N

Archangel

Daily Intention

I AM *Grateful for*

My Energy is directed ⟹

-------------------------➤
-------------------------➤
-------------------------➤
-------------------------➤
-------------------------➤
-------------------------➤
-------------------------➤
-------------------------➤
-------------------------➤

Act of Kindness

for yourself & others

Affirmation

Energy Check

Am I GROUNDED?　　Y / N　Y / N

Am I HYDRATED?　　Y / N　Y / N

Am I NOURISHED?　　Y / N　Y / N

Archangel

Daily Intention

I AM *Grateful for*

My Energy is directed →

Act of *Kindness*

for yourself & others

Affirmation

Energy Check

Am I GROUNDED?   Y / N   Y / N

Am I HYDRATED?   Y / N   Y / N

Am I NOURISHED?   Y / N   Y / N

Archangel

Daily Intention

I AM *Grateful for*

My Energy is directed ⇒

- ------------------➤
- ------------------➤
- ------------------➤
- ------------------➤
- ------------------➤
- ------------------➤
- ------------------➤
- ------------------➤
- ------------------➤

Energy Check

Am I GROUNDED?   Y / N   Y / N

Am I HYDRATED?   Y / N   Y / N

Am I NOURISHED?   Y / N   Y / N

Act of *Kindness*

for yourself & others

Affirmation

Archangel

Daily Intention

I AM *Grateful for*

My Energy is directed →

- - - - - - - - - - - - - ▶
- - - - - - - - - - - - - ▶
- - - - - - - - - - - - - ▶
- - - - - - - - - - - - - ▶
- - - - - - - - - - - - - ▶
- - - - - - - - - - - - - ▶
- - - - - - - - - - - - - ▶
- - - - - - - - - - - - - ▶
- - - - - - - - - - - - - ▶

Energy Check

Am I GROUNDED?   Y / N   Y / N

Am I HYDRATED?   Y / N   Y / N

Am I NOURISHED?   Y / N   Y / N

Act of *Kindness*

for yourself & others

Affirmation

Archangel
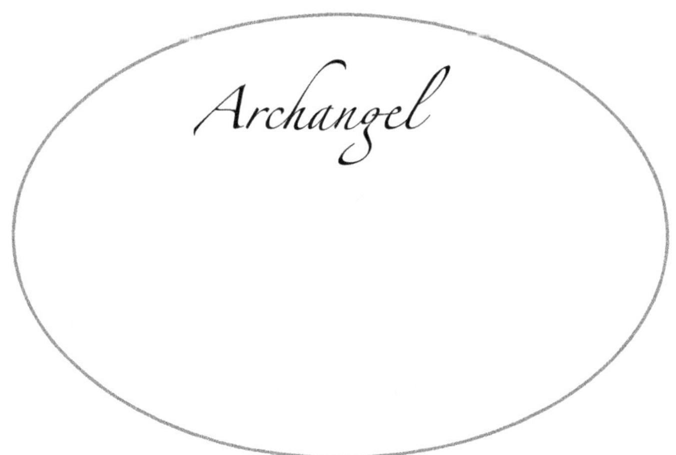

Daily Intention

I AM *Grateful for*

My Energy is directed

Act of *Kindness*

for yourself & others

Affirmation

Energy Check

Am I GROUNDED?   Y / N   Y / N

Am I HYDRATED?   Y / N   Y / N

Am I NOURISHED?   Y / N   Y / N

Archangel

Daily Intention

I AM *Grateful for*

My Energy is directed

- - - - - - - - - - - - - - - ▸
- - - - - - - - - - - - - - - ▸
- - - - - - - - - - - - - - - ▸
- - - - - - - - - - - - - - - ▸
- - - - - - - - - - - - - - - ▸
- - - - - - - - - - - - - - - ▸
- - - - - - - - - - - - - - - ▸
- - - - - - - - - - - - - - - ▸
- - - - - - - - - - - - - - - ▸

Energy Check

Am I GROUNDED?   Y / N   Y / N

Am I HYDRATED?   Y / N   Y / N

Am I NOURISHED?   Y / N   Y / N

Act of Kindness

for yourself & others

Affirmation

Archangel

Daily Intention

I AM *Grateful for*

My Energy is directed

Act of *Kindness*

for yourself & others

Affirmation

Energy Check

Am I GROUNDED?   Y / N   Y / N

Am I HYDRATED?   Y / N   Y / N

Am I NOURISHED?   Y / N   Y / N

Archangel

Daily Intention

I AM Grateful for

My Energy is directed

Act of Kindness

for yourself & others

Affirmation

Energy Check

Am I GROUNDED?   Y / N   Y / N

Am I HYDRATED?   Y / N   Y / N

Am I NOURISHED?   Y / N   Y / N

Archangel

The *Divine Mother*

Devotion & Unconditional Nurturing

Please note your experience with this Angelic Being:

What message does this energy bring?

What sights, sounds, feelings, thoughts, scents & emotions come to you?

What particular color, number or symbol has been brought to your awareness?

Affirmation & Intention

AFFIRMATIVE POWER: Affirmations are so powerful; when we commit to a particular thought or vibrational wave of thinking or feeling we bring that very frequency match into our reality & surroundings. This is true for positive or negative waves. This is why positive thinking is a golden tool. By speaking or thinking in the affirmative you are anchoring in the wish, idea or desired positive outcome or imprint on or of a given situation. It's being proactive vs. reactive in your life. Use the 21 day sheets for this exact idea.

MORNING AFFIRM: ***I am open* to receiving all of the abundance that the Universe is ready to deliver to me! I am worth it!***

(Repeat affirmation three times every morning. May I suggest arms wide open ready to receive)?

Dreams are experiences in other dimensions. When you have a vivd dream, that seems real, it is. It happened

Daily TIP: Set an alarm on your phone to remind you to call in your Angels throughout the day!

Archangels are omnipresent. They can be everywhere, at once. More than one place at time.

You have nothing to "learn". You are here to experience, through choice. Your choices. You are here to have the experiences that you create. You are the creator of your reality, at every level. The deep you seek within, the more of that knowledge you will uncover and remember.

Sacred Soak

Water is liquid Light.   The healing properties of Water are incredibly powerful. Taking a bath immersed in Water is an ultimate healing experience for your body.   I would love for you to you use Himalayan Salt in your Sacred Soaks, it's the pink salt that you can get at many health food stores in bulk. Be sure to select a fine grain version so it dissolves quickly and more thoroughly. This specific salt has a striking similarity in properly value, to amniotic fluid when it is mixed with Water. The salt helps to removes unwanted energies that we've picked up. It really clears the energy body and the physical body at the same time.

Essential oils are a wonderful addition to a sacred bath. I love flower oils, especially roses, so I often add a few drops of several varieties of floral essential oils in my baths and on my body, some oils art meant to go straight on the body though. Do your research if you are very sensitive or have known allergies. Lavender is great for relaxation. I most like to use Cedarwood and Evergreen, or any wood if I'm really feeling air headed or spacey, these woody elements help me to get super duper grounded and anchored in. You can grab a nice inexpensive essential oil to add to your bath from most of the same types of healthy market stores that carry the pink salt as well as item such as incense and intention candles. Enjoy burning nice incense, like Nag Champa for clearing, while you enjoy your Sacred Soak. Turn on some music that inspires your Heart, or relaxes your Soul. Sound is a healing tool, I use music to when I do energetic house clearings, music can change the vibration in a room within an instant. The idea is to create a Sacred Space for you to regenerate & recalibrate.

Soak with the intention of clearing all that no longer serves you. I ask you to invite Water to cleanse and clarify your entire being; Mind, Body and Soul. Ask your bath to carry any negativities or energy that does not serve you, down the drain. Release and surrender all your worries to be transmuted to LOVE.

Take this time to relax your mind and be present with your Sacred Soak. Feel the water, smell the incense, hear the music and listen for the Angels.

Anytime, morning, afternoon or night, a Sacred Soak can shift everything to tranquility & balance in an instant.

If you do not have a bathtub, you can have a Sacred Soak as well. Grant yourself a Sacred Foot Soak! Fill a large bowl or tub with your salt and oils, light your incense and you're all set.

Make it a point to connect with Water in this way DAILY. Especially though hydration, water is   key element to healing, and intuitive connection & growth.

Connect with Mother

Go outside. Put your feet in the grass. Walk in the sand. Hug a tree. Admire the beauty of a chatty songbird. Feel the sun on your face or the rain on your tongue. Make a snow angel. Take a hike or a stroll. Eat organic root vegetables. Stand under a waterfall.

Honor your appreciation for Mother Earth, and for Nature. Connect with her. This is *grounding*; this is how we stay connected to this planet and her energy. When we are grounded, we are present. When we are present we are aware. When we are aware we receive GIFTS. This awareness serves you very well, so I suggest you go get grounded. As you connect with Mother, ask her to help you release any personal motherly wounds that may harbor within you, about yourself or your own mothers and grandmothers. Release the guilt you feel about your current situation. Ask the Divine Mother to nurture you in a way you've always desired and deserved. Let us all feel the Love and Comfort of the Divine Mother within. Ask and allow all mother emotions, resentments and fears be dissolved into the Earth to be returned into Love.

The Archangels work very closely with the energy spirit of the Animal & Plant Kingdoms. You will begin to identify Archangels teaming up with certain animals on a regular basis. Same with Flower essence, Crystals & Minerals, too. Everything is inter-connected, you will find that it all leads back to you. Regardless of the path or tools. You always find your way. You will be guided to them by your Angels.

Dailey Invocation Samples

Archangel RAPHAEL: Body & Health

Dearest Archangel Raphael, I honor your presence & thank you for infusing your Emerald Green Rays into every cell of my being. Please assist in my healing, the disconnection and reconnection of body and mind. Assist me to speak, and to listen to my physical body to answer. Raphael, help bring me to clarity along my path to self-healing. Thank you, Archangel Raphael.

Take a moment and listen to your body. What guidance are you receiving from it? What is Raphael telling you about your body & your healing? Listen to your body, it has a message for you. Make friends with your body, have a journaling sessions & conversation with Body.

Archangel MICHAEL: Security & Protection

Dearest Archangel Michael, I am honored to have your presence with & within me. Surround me fully in your Deep Blue energetic vibration. Please allow me to remember I am safe and protected at all times. Michael, please remove all energies & entities so only those that serve my highest and best good remain. Let go of all else. Thank yo, Thank you. Thank you.

Relax, breath & feel the connection with Michael, what guidance does he/she bring you?

What feeling or thoughts are coming up for you?

Archangel ZADKIEL: Transmutation & Forgiveness

My Dear Archangel Zadkiel, Please immerse me in your essence of mercy and deep compassion. Allowing for all hurts and old wounds to be mended and healed. I ask the Violet Flame of Transmutation to filter in and transmute all guilts and shames into Love. Thank you for your everlasting forgiveness, Zadkiel.

Write &/or contemplate about what comes up for you when you connect with this loving Angel. These are feelings, changes and emotions that are waiting to be healed within.

Archangel CHAMUEL: Unconditional & Self-Love

My Dear and Divine Archangel Chamuel, shower me with your vibrant Pink Ray Energy. I appreciate you surrounding all my situations in Pure Perfect Love. Thank you for the clarity to love myself first and foremost. Chamuel I adore you, for reminding me to adore myself. I am Love. I am Loved, and so it is.

How are you feeling as you connect with Chamuel's energy ? What comes up within your Heart Chakra?

(As we move forward we will touch on the Chakra System & the Angel Connection, along with Dowsing the Chakra for healing!)

I like to be reminded to call in the Angels on a consistent & regular basis. When I do it on a routine basis, I stay much more committed to the process. The 7 days of the week are a great way to stay connected. Here are a few daily intentions and invocations for your Angelic toolbox. Setting daily intention for gas personal and business is also a great way to co-create your reality with precision. Here are some very basic ideas to use and expand upon.

MONDAY intention

My Dearest Archangels, thank you for surrounding me with your Light, Wisdom, and Comfort today, and everyday and so it is.

Find yourself in a space of Peace in the morning, no computer or phone. Just be present with your morning. Breathe......

TUESDAY intention

My Dearest Archangels, thank you for helping me see clearly the Courage, Strength, Beauty and Love within myself and all things.

Lying in your bed, is a sacred space. Call in your Angels and the energy of Abundance before you even get out of bed. Receive... Breathe...... Open your arms wide, take deep breathes in your chest and invite the energy into your Heart.

WEDNESDAY intention

My Dearest Archangels, thank you for assisting me with your presence. I let go of all that no longer serves me, my family or the highest good of ALL. I am Freedom and so it is.

Create a quiet space of tranquility for yourself. Remember, no computer or phone. Just be present with your morning. Breathe...

THURSDAY intention

My Dearest Divine Archangels, I honor you. I create within your colorful & radiant energies. Thank you for the assistant to sing, dance, paint, & create with soulful passion.

Create a sacred space of rhythm for yourself, play some music, listen to birds. Be present with you and your morning. Breathe...... Create....

FRIDAY intention

Archangels, I adore you. Your Light brings Clarity of my Vision, my Dreams. Along with the Clarity, & Clearing of vibrational frequency. Thank you or your assistance to see clearly my path ahead.

I AM.

A sacred soak in the bath is a great way to start a beautiful day. . Call upon your Angels and Guides to pour beauty over you. Flow and Allow the healing powers of Water to assist you to clarify your self.

Angels can bring their energy & essence through people in your physical world, to bring you a message. It's usually quite obvious, there's a certain twinkle in the eye when a concentrated dose of Archangel energy presents itself in this way.

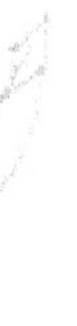

*Feather wands are a favorite tool of mine for clearing energy. I love to indulge in my Shamanism. I use a hawk & turkey feather to clear the energetic field around myself, my clients, my kids & my pets. When yo can no turn or use scented clearing tools the feather **wand** is a must!*

SATURDAY intention

__Mighty Archangels of the Highest Order. Your presence is appreciated. Allow my Heart to be Free Spirited & Childlike. I am Joy.__

Create your quiet sacred space for yourself anywhere. Listen to music. Just be present with yourself and your desire for JOY in all areas of your life. Breathe...

SUNDAY intention

__Mighty Archangels of the Highest Order. Your presence is appreciated. Allow my Heart to be Free Spirited & Childlike. I am Joy.__

Create your quiet sacred space for yourself anywhere. Listen to music. Just be present with your morning. Breathe…

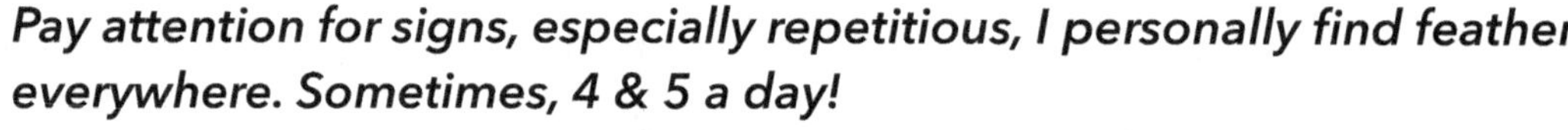

Pay attention for signs, especially repetitious, I personally find feather everywhere. Sometimes, 4 & 5 a day!

Most Angels, and especially Archangels have a great send of humor and fun! Tap into that childlike part of yourself when it's time to play!

The Archangels speak to me in color, often. I see color with my clairvoyance and I see color in my physical world. A spilled can of purple paint is clearly I sign from the Violet Flame, and Archangel Zadkiel. I'd be calling Zadkiel in for a conversation for sure!

I sometimes I use dice, flash cards and whatever is available as a tool for divining. I enclose can act as a pendulum in a pinch. I love Oracle Cards , they are one of my favorites, too!

21 Days of Archangels

MONDAY	TUESDAY	WEDNESDAY	THURSDAY	FRIDAY	SATURDAY	SUNDAY

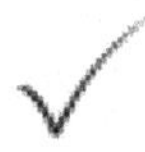 Place check marks in the box when you have connected with and called in your Angels for the day. Use multiple check marks to show how often you've brought your awareness to the Angelic Realm that particular day.

 Place hearts in the appropriate box, when you receive guidance, healing or clarity from your Angels. Look for the SIGNS

Pendulum & Dowsing Divination

* Clear your pendulum. Anything can be used a s pendulum as long as it has a distinct form of motion, swing. Clear using sunlight, moonlight, salt bath, or your own breath.

* Program your pendulum, Meaning give it instructions. " You will assist me in the communication of truth in the highest good all."

* Get yourself nicely present, grounded & centered. Check your emotions, be sure your clear to channel.

* Call in your Spiritual Team of advisers & guides whenever you connect & channel energy. While also surrounding yourself with Light & Safety.

* Ask your pendulum to show you it's 'yes & no', and also 'maybe'.

* Ask permission to have a conversation using this pendulum as your tool to assist you to channel the energy necessary.

* ASK YOUR QUESTIONS . Be precise & clear. You make use a chart or any other from of dowsing map. Just be clear, yes & no's are great for that. I use dowsing for so many things. Simple yes or no's that I'm stuck on. The akashic record work I do, Soul Realignment, is where I use the pendulum a great deal. I have provided you several dowsing charts in this experience.

* **You must step out of the way! You can not be emotionally attached and get accuracy with a pendulum or as an intuitive.** If you are having trouble, ask an Angel for assistance in getting out of the way .

Archangel 101 Dowsing Charts

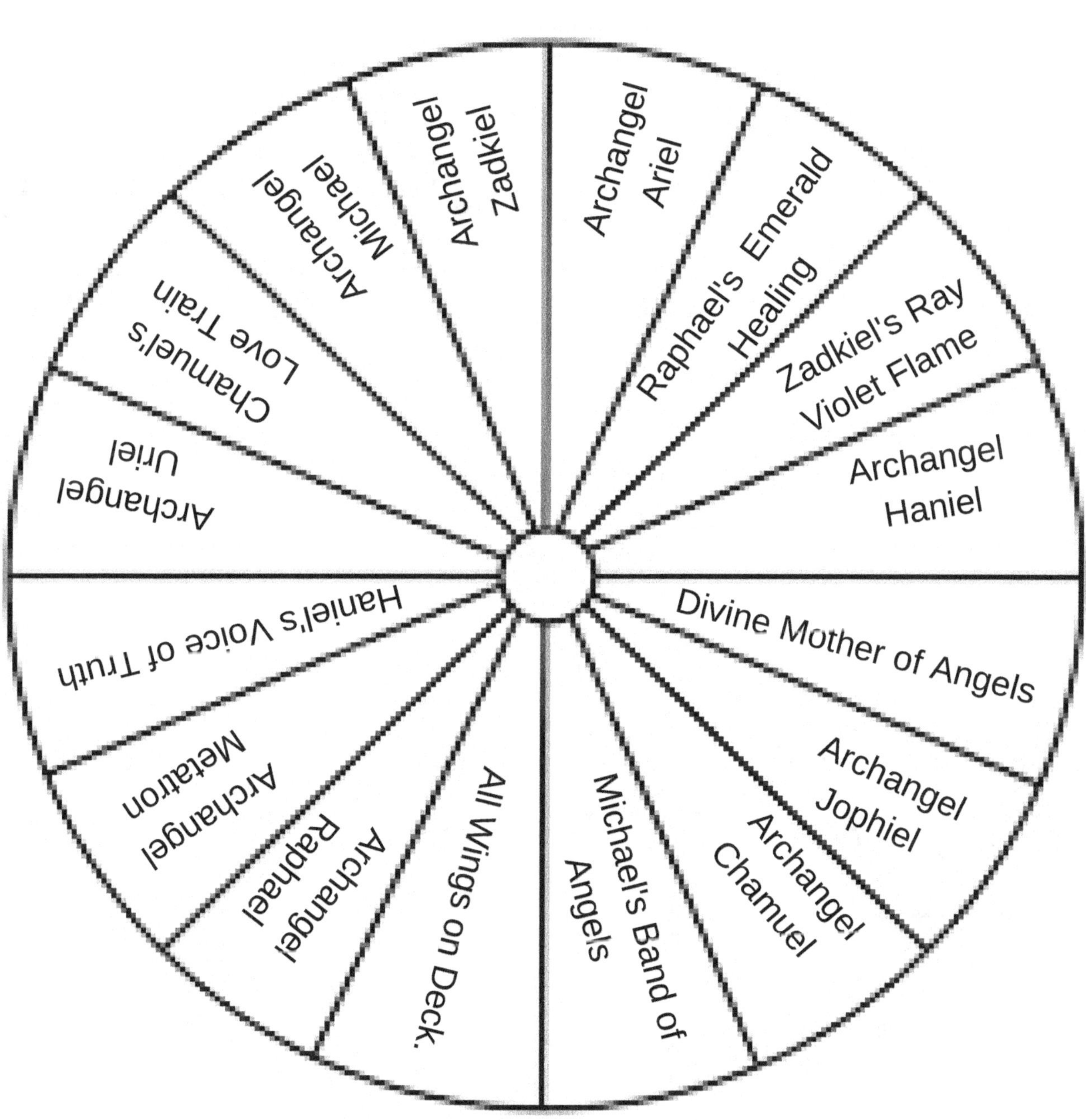

Dowsing Charts & Maps

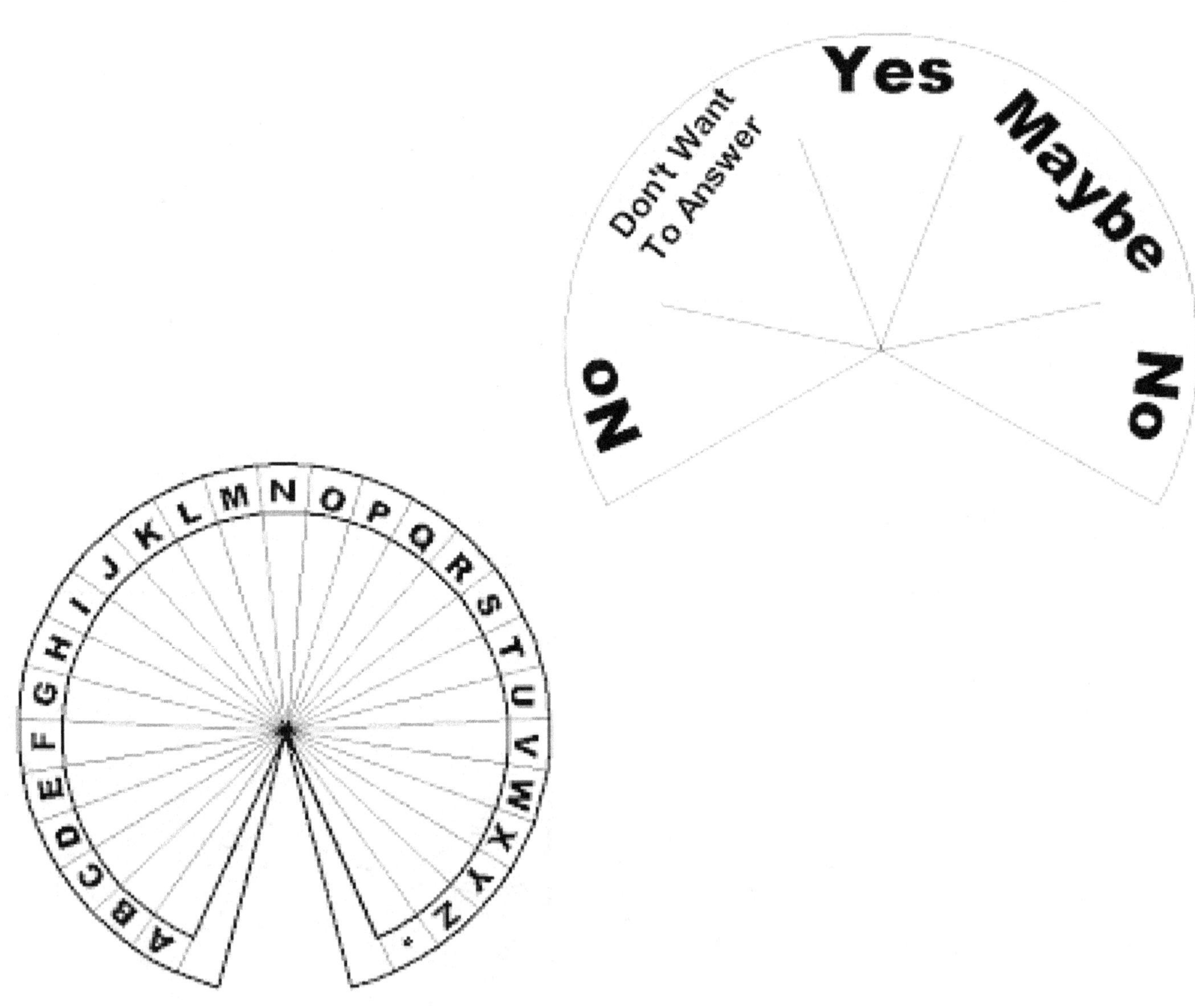

Intuitive Gifts & Strengths Chart

Using your pendulum, asking Y/N to see if you are open to each Claire, yet. You can even dowse to put them in order of strength. Ask to identify your primary and secondary. You can also use this chart to ask about the best way to communicate with particular Angels & Guides.

Clairvoyance (clear seeing)

Clairsentience (clear physical feeling)

Claircognizance (clear knowing)

Clairtangency (clear touching)

Clairaudience (clear hearing)

Clairsalience (clear smelling)

Clairempathy (clear emotional feeling)

Clairgustance (clear tasting)

CROWN- **Violet/White**~Connection & Knowingness: GABRIEL

THIRD EYE- **Indigo** ~ Clarity of Vision: MICHAEL

THROAT- **Blue** ~ Speaking Your Truth: HANIEL

HEART – **Green/Pink** Center ~ Love & Healing: RAPHAEL & CHAMUEL

SOLAR PLEXUS- **Yellow** ~ Personal Power & Courage: ARIEL

SACRAL- **Orange** ~ Manifestation & Creation: JOPHIEL

ROOT – **Red** ~ Grounding & Nurturing: URIEL

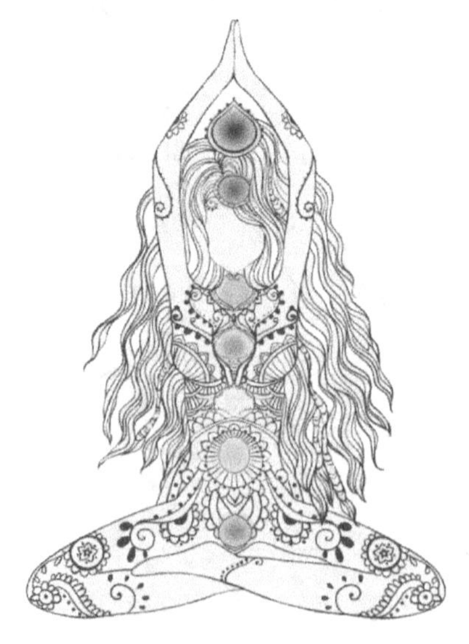

Chakra Dowsing & Balancing

Use your pendulum to check for imbalance. Use this information to call in the appropriate Archangel to assist you or your client in healing & balancing this chakra. Your intention alone, to balance & harmonize the chakra is enough to shift the energy into place. Ask Metatron to assist ...

Hold pendulum over each chakra one by one, on the chart

or in person. Ask your pendulum to show you if the chakra is spinning in the appropriate direction. All chakra spin clock-wise, except for male energy, and their crown chakra is opposite, counter clockwise, when harmonized. Check each one see if it is clockwise, with that one exception. Identify which chakra need to be cleared & balanced. OR simply ask YES or NO's like 'Does the Crown Chakra need balanced?' This can help you pinpoint pain for yourself, family member, child, or client. Dowsing is a great way to get information in a succinct way. Pendulum use for emotional answers & mediumship are a little more tricky. **You** can sway the pendulum. You must be complete out of the way or attached to outcome to have accuracy

with dowsing using a pendulum.

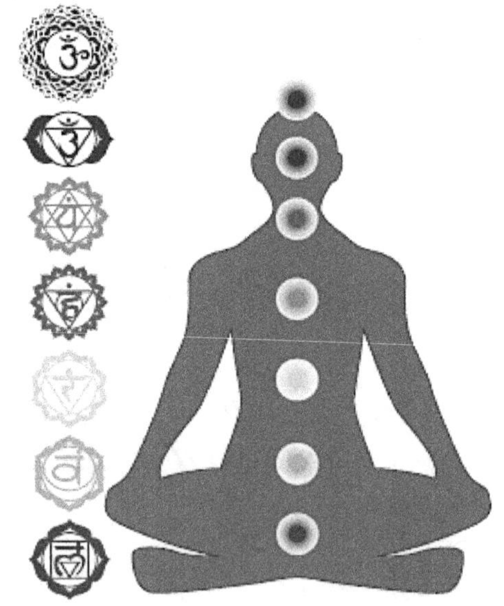

Reading & Clarity Sheet

INTENTION: State your intention for your dowsing & channeling session. Call in your White Light and any of your Team Members you'd like to invoke. Get centered & clear.

What is the concern? or question? **Be clear.**

Use Archangel Dowsing Charts to identify present situation details.

Angelic Guides best suited to assist are:

<u>Primary Archangel :</u>

<u>Secondary Archangel assist:</u>

<u>Additional:</u>

(Ask if there is a Secondary & Additional, use "yes" & "no" with your pendulum for this.)

<u>Chakra Involved:</u>

CROWN   THIRD-EYE   THROAT   HEART   SOLAR.PLEXUS   SACRAL   ROOT

(Use Chakra System Dowsing Chart to identify. Asking "yes" or "no" if each Chakra is balanced properly, & which need attention or are con-tributing to the issue. You may use your dowsing charts to assist.)

<u>Is clearing necessary for this Chakra ?</u> **Y N**

<u>Is this an ongoing issue ?</u> **Y N**

<u>Is more work to be done to uncover the root cause or trigger?</u> **Y N**

(If Yes to chakra clearing, then you can clear it yourself.

 Start by imagining and directing the chakra to turn in the appropriate di-rection. While you infuse the essence of energy that is the color match to that Chakra. You can visualize in your minds eye or use your hands to give energy in person. All the while, asking the Primary & Angelic team to as-sist. Infuse the color until You get a No answer on clearing. then you will know you are complete with the clearing. If it's more of an ongoing or much deeper issue then you may need to work that Chakra for a few days, or a week or so. Use your charts and ask questions that lead you to clear picture of what is needed for what is going on on an energetic level.)

Additional information :

> What Color is associated with the Healing needed most at this time?
>
> **RED ORANGE YELLOW GREEN PINK BLUE INDIGO VIOLET/WHITE**

(Use your charts & Guidebook to identify the Archangel & Chakra by the colors revealed.)

Create your own Yes, No & Maybe questions & keep track below. This will help you get super clear and accurate during your self or client session.

Y N M
Y N M
Y N M
Y N M
Y N M
Y N M
Y N M
Y N M
Y N M

Angel & Guide Conversation Sheet

Intention:

State your intention for your dowsing & channeling session. Call in your White Light and any of your Team Members you'd like to invoke. Get centered & clear.

What is the concern? or question? Purpose of connection?

(You may choose to invoke a particular Angel or just see who shows up!)

***ALWAYS ask if the entity or being you are communicating with is "OF LIGHT". Require A "YES" answer or DO NOT move forward.**

***Surround yourself with Michael Blue Energy for extra protection along with your White Light Bubble of Protection.**

Use Archangel Dowsing Charts to identify present situation details.

Identify Conversation:

<u>Primary Archangel :</u>

<u>Other Guides?</u> Y N

(Use A-Z dowsing chart to identify names of other guides in the conversation.)

<u>How Many ?</u> 1 2 3

(I'd put a limit on the number of peeps in the conversation. Start a new

conversation with each guide if necessary)

<u>Chakra Involved:</u> Y N

CROWN   THIRD-EYE   THROAT   HEART   SOLAR.PLEXUS   SACRAL   ROOT

(Use Chakra System Dowsing Chart to identify. Asking "yes" or "no" if

each Chakra is balanced properly, & which need attention or are con-

tributing to the issue. You may use your dowsing charts to assist.)

<u>Is clearing necessary for this Chakra ?</u> **Y N**

<u>Is this an ongoing issue ?</u> **Y N**

<u>Is more work to be done to uncover the root cause or trigger?</u> **Y N**

(If Yes to chakra clearing, then you can clear it yourself.

 Start by imagining and directing the chakra to turn in the appropriate direction. While you infuse the essence of energy that is the color match to that Chakra. You can visualize in your minds eye or use your hands to give energy in person. All the while, asking the Primary & Angelic team to assist. Infuse the color until You get a No answer on clearing. then you will know you are complete with the clearing. If it's more of an ongoing or much deeper issue then you may need to work that Chakra for a few days, or a week or so. Use your charts and ask questions that lead you to clear picture of what is needed for what is going on on an energetic level.)

Is there a message using the alphabet chart? **Y N**

(If so, take this opportunity to use the A-Z dowsing chart to spell words of guidance from the Angelic Realm.)

Additional information :

What Color is associated with the Healing needed most at this time?

RED   ORANGE   YELLOW   GREEN   PINK   BLUE   INDIGO   VIOLET/WHITE

(Use your charts & Guidebook to identify the Archangel & Chakra by the colors revealed.)

Channeling Chart

INTENTION

CONNECTION

FINDINGS

Create your own Yes, No & Maybe questions for this Angel & keep track below. This will help you get super clear and accurate during your conversation & channeling session.

Y N M

Y N M

Y N M

Y N M

Y N M

Y N M

Y N M

Y N M

Y N M

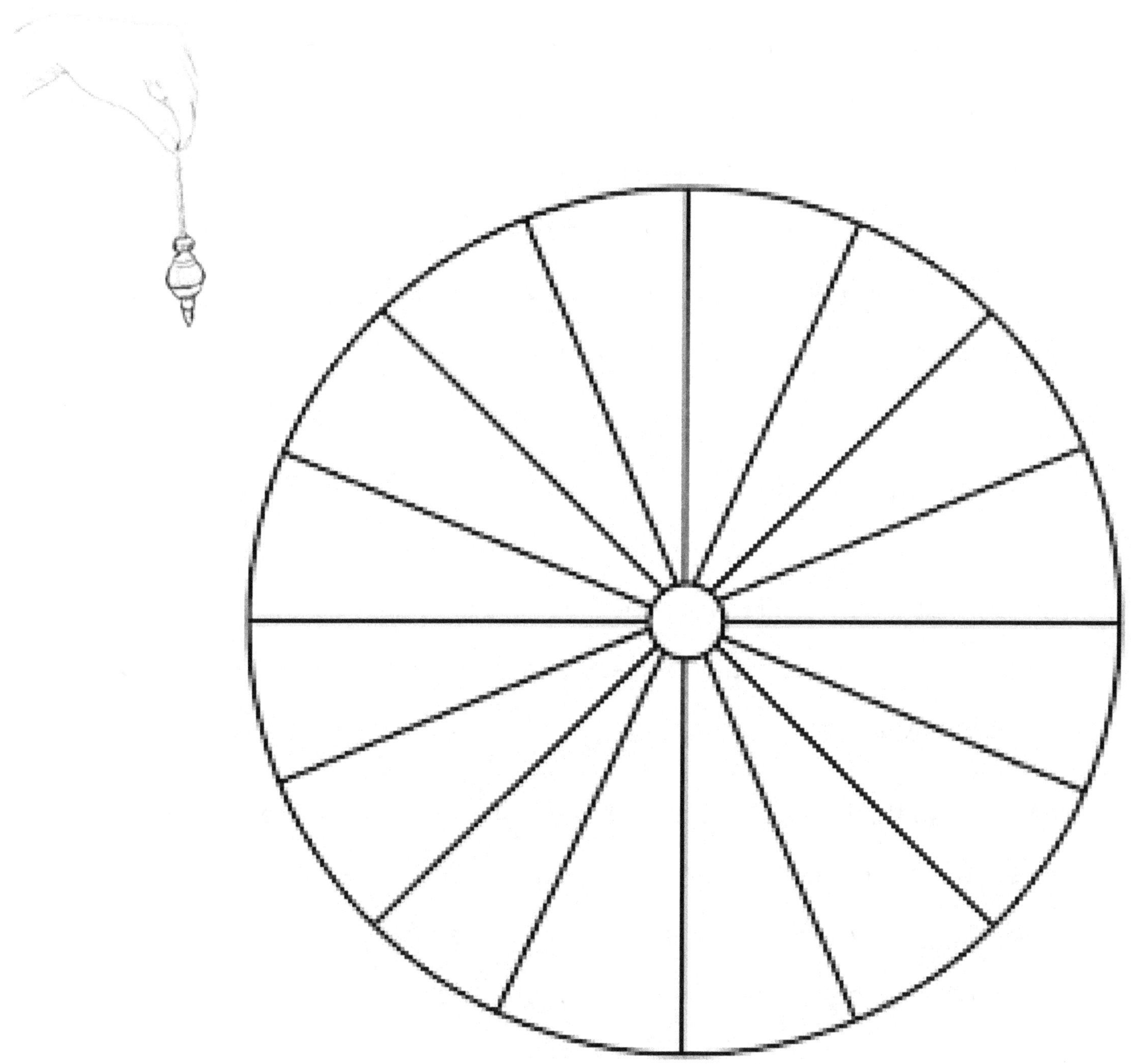

Journaling & Channeling

You will be prompted to enjoy in some journaling and note taking within this Course. Writing is a way of moving and clearing energy, as well as rock solid manifesting tool. It's a very important tool in the process. It is so important that there is a whole chapter of journaling & writing within this book. I have also provided space in the book for notes & doodles, I'm a doodle hound!I get messages trough doodle, art and what some would consider scribble. Look for it. Invocation & Intention

Calling in the energy of the Angels can be as elaborate & as simple as you desire. It's your language that you are communication with. Speak in a way that feels right for you. Journaling is fantastic for intention setting In turn, they will return that perfect communication style, easy for you to understand and recognize.

When you think about them, that's an invocation for their energy to be present. There are a number of ways to have conversations with the Angels. They may send you an image or picture in your mind, you may hear a song verse in your head, you may feel static or goosebumps in your physics body. You may see a license plate with the next part to your con-versation.

Here are a few examples on how to call in the energy. They may be spoken aloud or projected through thought. Call them in DAILY, or even HOURLY. You can not ask too much of these fantastic guides! There is no task that is too small or unimportant.

Please, ask for assistance, guidance & signs consistently and as often as necessary!

Channeling & Automatic Writing

Are you ready to expand through Angelic Communication?

Journaling with the Angels is a wonderful creative asset to add to your spiritual toolbox. Through journaling you are able to express energy, gain wisdom, receive guidance, and create awareness for yourself. There are many forms of journaling, all are perfect. Each unique style of journaling serves the individual. You may journal once a week, or maybe you journal on particular circumstances or you may be you're a daily journal junkie. The wonderful part about this is, it's your tool to utilize as YOU see fit.

Personally, writing things out helps me see them more clearly and helps me gain another perspective. I also use my writing to set intention for that in which I want to create. I also a big time doodler, can you relate? I love to draw and have realized that my doodles are healing, just like words. For this reason you will find plenty of doodle pages in your journal.

As I mentioned, there are many ways to journal & channel energy. Here are a few suggestions for you as you move through your process.

Automatic Writing: This form of journaling is fascinating to me. The first time I did it, I couldn't believe what's happening. In automatic writing, you get yourself complexity center through short meditation or prayer. Setting the intention to be the channel for the information to flow. Removing your own thoughts and simply opening up to the information and then allowing that information to automatically come through you, and onto the paper. I have provided you with a detailed example in the next few pages.

Clarity Journaling: It can sometimes (often times!) challenging to reach a point of clarity on our own circumstances. When we are knee deep into a challenge, it's a bit of a struggle to pull that leg to the next step with certainty. Setting the intention to receive guidance and clarity on a situation though journaling is very effective. It's like talking to a friend, it always helps to get it out and see it from their perspective. The ideas and confusion may be all tight and stuck, and talking it out can really help you see the details more clearly. Journaling is "talking it out".

Intention Journaling: Affirmation and intention arc important keys to co-creating in this world. Journaling can be used as a powerful way to set your intentions and affirm them on paper to bring your desires into manifestation.

Gratitude Journaling: Gratitude is a transformative energy that brings blessings and growth. When you take note and really count your blessings, your heart expands. Journaling can help you find the gold nugget in situations & circumstances that seem to be the most challenging. Setting your journaling intention on gratitude, will reveal the treasure of a rough experience.

Release Writing: Expressing emotion through journaling is very healing experience. Letting go of the dense energy stored within you through journaling, makes room for more LOVE and blessing. Lower vibrational energies like anger, guilt, & fear can be released from your energy field though journaling.

Diary Style: This type of journaling is all about reflection. It seems to be more of a freestyle way of writing. Normally, this entails looking back on your day and writing down the feelings and actions you have taken part in.

Remember your experience is uniquely perfect for you. You may choose to do a different style of journaling every time you crack open this simple but powerful little tool. There is no wrong way to walk you path, journaling included.

Throughout your inspirational journal you will find word prompts to use, if you feel guided. These can also be used as guidance, similar to oracle cards. Simply flip to a page and receive your message.

Automatic Writing Tip

Find yourself a very comfortable space and position to relax, that still allows you to be able to write. You will want to be sure to have your pen/pencil and journal at arms length.

Set your intention, with your thoughts, on the circumstance or topic that you wish to receive clarity on. You may even set this intention to auto write with a particular spirit guide or angelic being. Sending out the intention to open your heart to greater & grander experience & expressions of your truth.

Close your eyes and take several deep breaths. Breathing in peace & love, exhaling all that no longer serves your highest good. Relax your mind and give your body permission to rest, ask your cells to absorb all the peace & love filling your body through your breath. Surround yourself with a bubble pure white light. Once you feel completely relaxed, slowly open your eyes. Take your journal and begin writing in this very relaxed meditative state.

Allow the writing to take over, without conscious thought. Write or draw whatever comes. Do not judge the information or try to make sense of it. Complete sentences are not important. Keep writing without going back and reading until you have finished. Grammar and neatness to not matter at this point. Expect that the information will not make sense to you until you are complete and ready to translate it into your message. Let it flow through you. The idea is to get yourself out of the way.

You are the channel. Begin by setting your intentions below. List what you want to bring into your life. Make your Love List , things you would LOVE to bring into your life. What you REALLY desire to bring into your reality? How would you see your perfect world? Imagine what it would feel like and it will lead you to it.

LOVE LIST

Strength

Courage

Honor

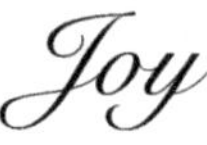

Joy

Peace

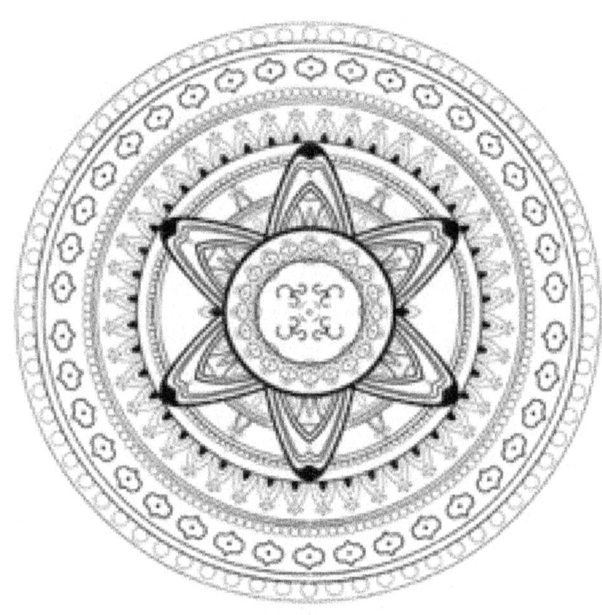

Boundaries

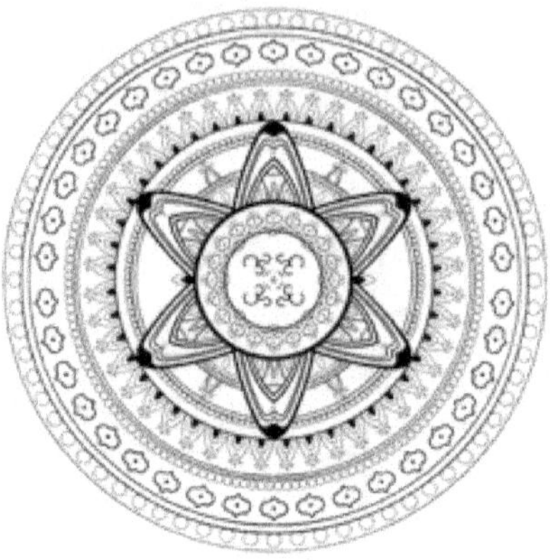

Patience

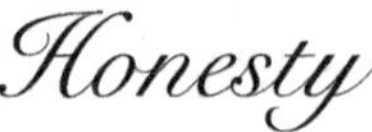

Honesty

Blessings

Growth

Receive

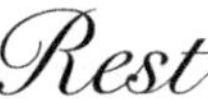# Rest

Breathe

Expand

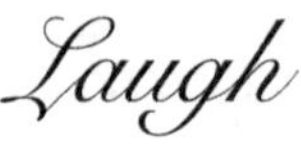

Dance

Transform

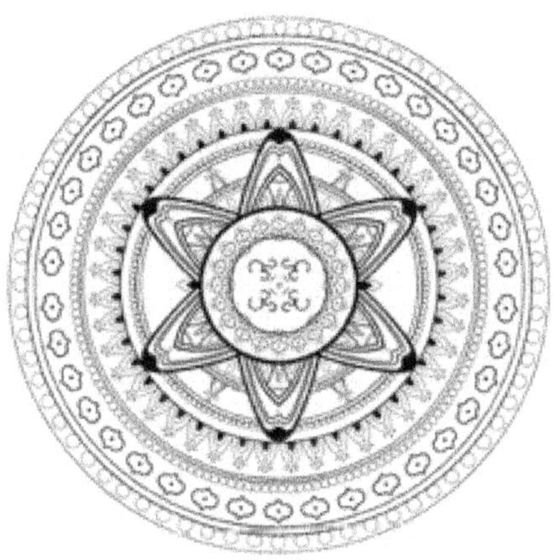

Resonate

Serve

Explore

Beauty

Divine Timing

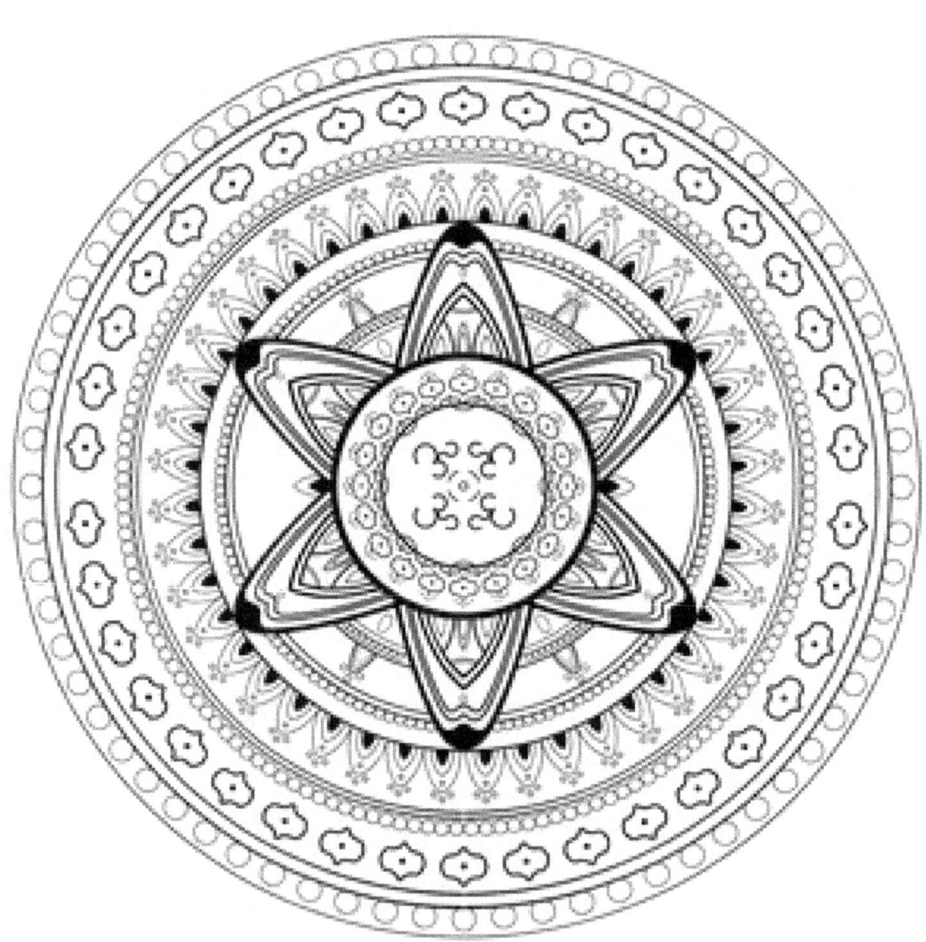

Ground

Humility

Freedom

Responsibility

Desire

Wealth

Wisdom

Passion

Peace

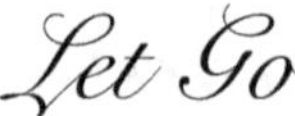

Let Go

Compassion

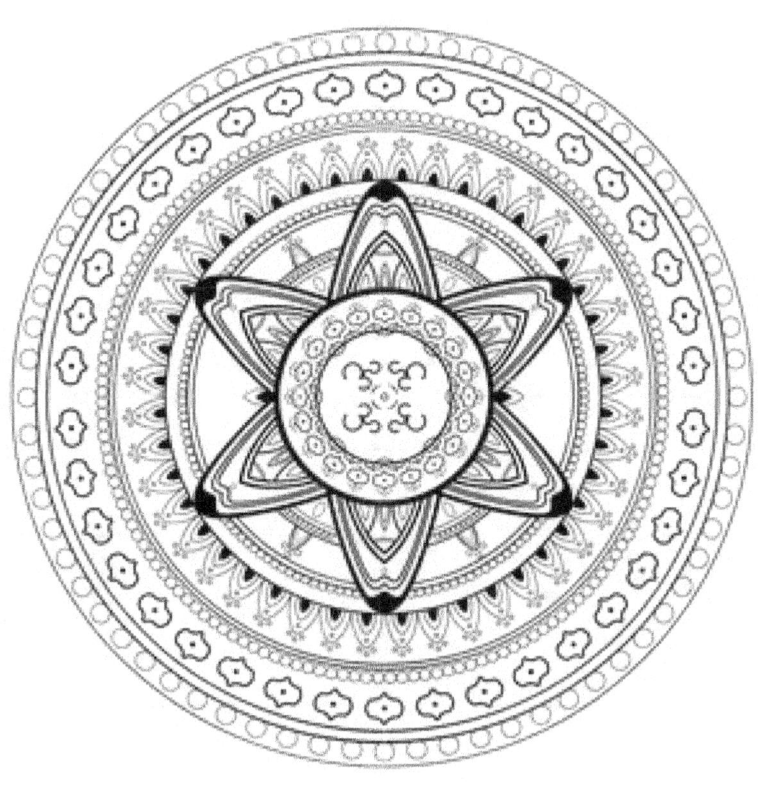

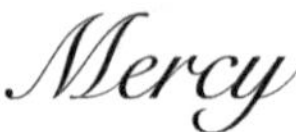

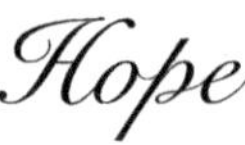

Hope

Heart

Soul

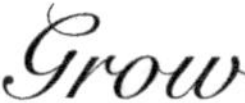

Grow

Learn

Discernment

Respect

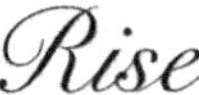

Rise

Truth

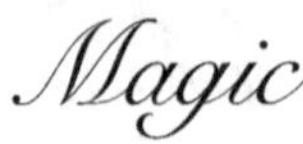

Magic

Success

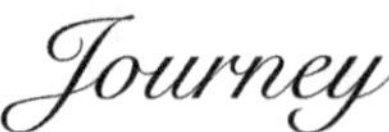

Journey

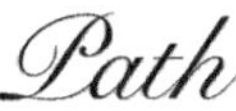

Path

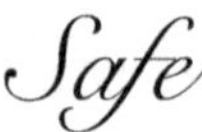

Safe

Retreat

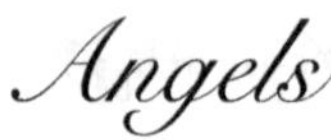

Angels

Soul Family

Cherish

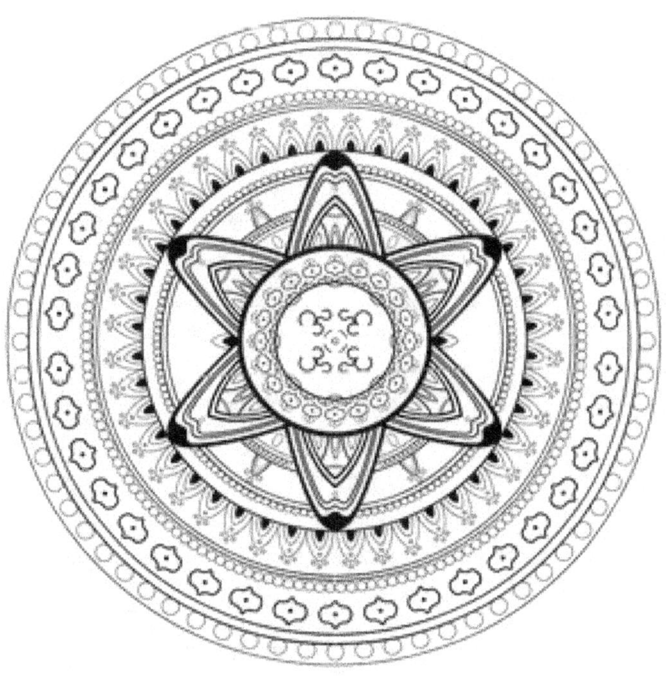

Integrity

Motivation

Gratitude

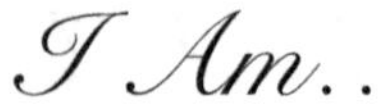

I Am...

Notes & Doodles

Daily Intention

I AM Grateful for

My Energy is directed

Act of Kindness

for yourself & others

Affirmation

Energy Check

Am I GROUNDED?   Y / N   Y / N

Am I HYDRATED?   Y / N   Y / N

Am I NOURISHED?   Y / N   Y / N

Archangel

Archangel ___________

Channeling Chart

INTENTION

CONNECTION

FINDINGS

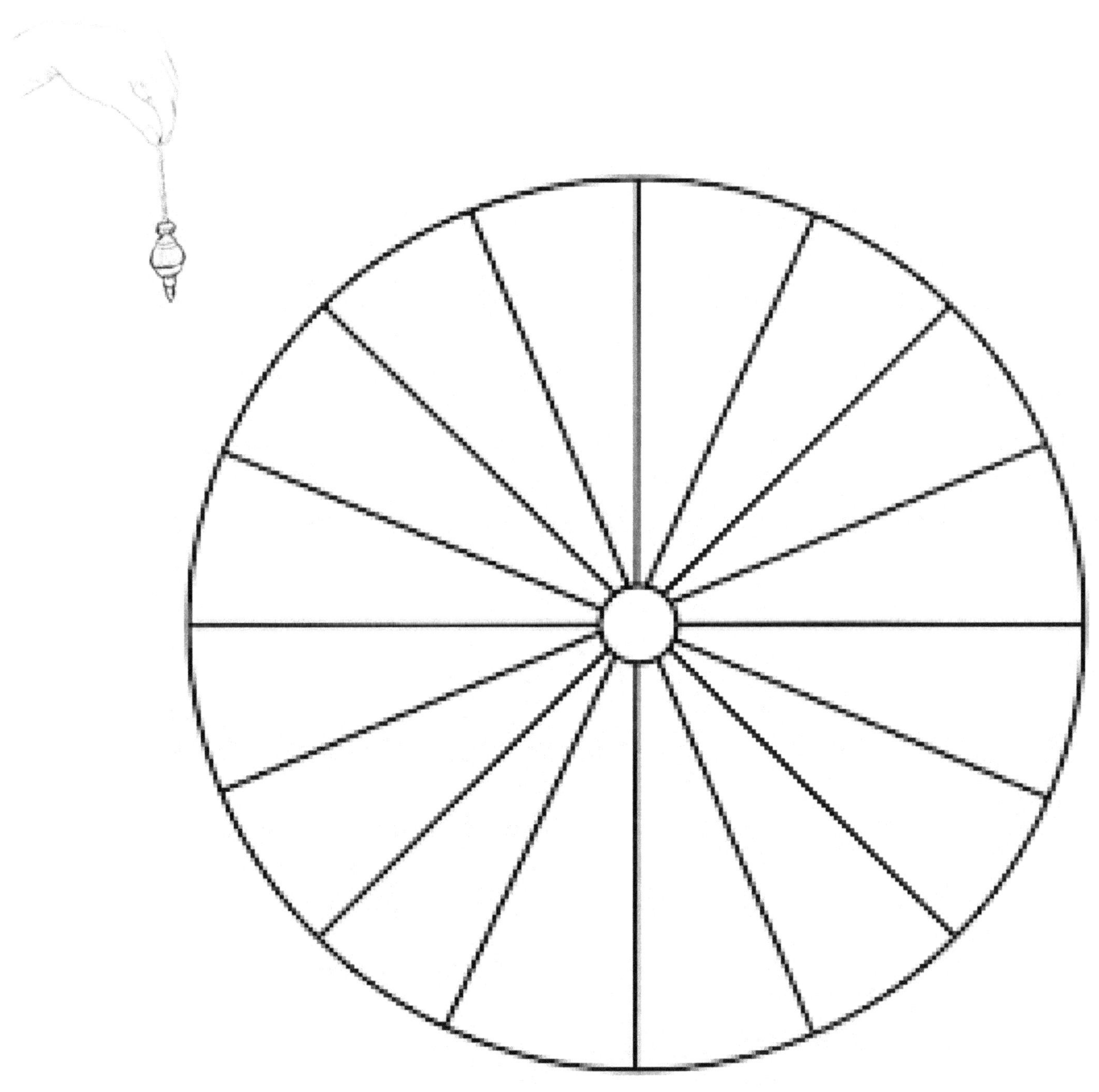

Notes & Doodles

MONDAY	TUESDAY	WEDNESDAY	THURSDAY	FRIDAY	SATURDAY	SUNDAY

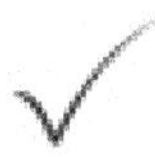 Place check marks in the box when you have connected with and called in your Angels for the day. Use multiple check marks to show how often you've brought your awareness to the Angelic Realm that particular day.

 Place hearts in the appropriate box, when you receive guidance, healing or clarity from your Angels. Look for the SIGNS

Notes & Doodles

Notes & Doodles

Notes & Doodles

Notes & Doodles

Notes & Doodles

Notes & Doodle

Personal Sessions, VIP Retreats & More

www.lisanicole.net

AVAILABLE AT

www.lisanicole.net

Questions, Comments & Experiences

lisanicole@lisanicole.net

Thank you, Angels.